THE TRUTH ABOUT WEIGHT LOSS & DIETS

A Proven System Which Never Fails

I0408482

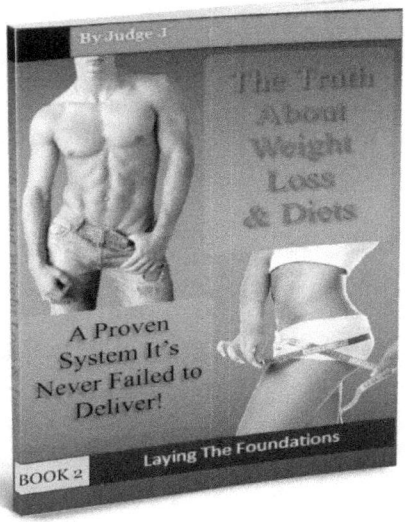

By: JUDGE J

This book came to life, because of my need to spread the truth about **'Weight Loss',** and to dispel the _**MYTHS**_ that surrounds this subject. This book is based on actual experiences, trial and error, gathered between my students and I, over the last 50yrs. I guarantee if you follow the advice echoed in this book you will SUCCEED! More about the Author visit... http://increasemusclesize.net

INTRODUCTION

Why Diets Don't Work

I have been writing this book for over a year now, and it's taken me this long, because I wanted to get the balance right between helping the ordinary everyday person who doesn't train in the gym, to lose fat and maintain their lifestyle.

I also want to help the guy who trains in the gym, training with weights, to reach their ripped body goals.

Over the years, I have seen so many new diets, fitness, and bodybuilding fads, come and go.

It's made me furious, because most are written by people who have never had to diet, or set foot in a gym.

These so called experts are conning the public with their lies and misconceptions.

They know nothing about the self-sacrifice, heartaches, blood, sweat and tears involved with burning away body fat. Dieters, fitness coaches, and those who trainer with weights, put themselves through hell in the hope of reaching their desired body goals?

It's **NOT** your fault, because they use doctored photos and false testimonials, to help lure people aboard, and use every trick in the book to take money from the pockets of people who really do need their help.

The book shops have shelves full of failed diets, what does that tell you about the nature of diets...***they don't work***!

So, I decided to write this book to help inform you, the reader, of the honest, truth, and proven weight loss facts, behind diets.

I have been involved in the fitness game for over **50**yrs; I learnt my lessons through the hard knock school of life, during my school days, my martial arts, and bodybuilding career.

I see people, daily, pushing themselves hard through their routines trying to reach their goals, but failing, because they are unwittingly taking the advice of someone who they believe knows what they are talking about... it makes my blood boil.

This book is dedicated to those who want to learn *'How'* to lose body fat, and maintain their desired weight levels for the rest of their life.

It doesn't matter whether or not, you go to the gym, or you are a house-wife, like to keep fit, or build muscle mass, we ALL have the same goals, to burn off body fat, then control and maintain that position.

It's my personal belief and experiences, that's lead me to understand that those lessons I learnt in the gym, through blood, sweat, and tears, following in the footsteps of successful competitors, can, and will help you burn off your body fat too.

This knowledge can be used by anyone, wishing to gain some weight management skills.

When it comes to losing and managing weight, there really is no difference between the needs of the general public, and those of a weight-trainer, except the levels they wish to reach.

The real trick about losing and managing your weight is knowledge.

You will learn that knowledge as you read through the pages of this book. After, you will have a road-map to follow.

This knowledge will help you to both lose body fat, and maintain your weight, for as long as you wish to follow it.

The journey will be long and hard, but coupled with the lessons you learnt in my first book *'How to lose and maintain your weight'*... http://mybooksupply.com/wp/lose-weight-diet-for-life ... you can, and will succeed.

Visit my website to check my book out: http://mybooksupply.com

How to Succeed Where Others Have Failed

I guess I'm quizzed about diets almost daily; people always want to know **'how'** to either lose weight or increase their muscle size.

Unfortunately, it's not as simple as you may think, after all, if it were then my gym would be full to the rafters with people losing weight, and obesity would be extinct.

Believe it or not, but a whopping **95%** of those people who go on a diet will fail?

'Yes', and not only will they regain their original body weight, but they will go on to pile on even more body fat.

One thing that's very clear, you can't take body fat off overnight, it takes time...months, maybe years in fact!

When I think of a diet for one of my members, I'm not going to give them the type of diet the public try, why?

Because today's diets are restrictive, they are unhealthy, and very confusing…they are totally unrealistic and plainly just don't work.

There's no doubt that this is a vast subject, and many people find it extremely difficult to lose, or put on body mass.

Having said that, there is a glimmer of hope for us all, but it will require you to take a leap of faith and change your life-style…**are you ready**?

I will endeavour to do my very best to keep this book as basic, and as simple to understand as I can… no bullshit, just plain simple talking.

Anyway, even if you didn't want to lose or put on any body weight, there is some very interesting research going on that suggests and confirms an old idea.

That reducing calories has some very beneficial side effects, more on this later, well worth sticking through to the end of this book.

Putting on weight or losing weight can be categorized by one very simple truth, if you consume more calories than your body can burn off, then the end result will be **'overweight'**… that my friends is a fact!

The same, of course, works in the opposite way, if you are burning off more calories than you are eating…***you will lose weight.***

I get people constantly telling me that it doesn't matter how much they diet they can't lose weight.

Or they eat next- to-nothing… try telling that to someone starving in some third world country who looks like a skeleton.

I personally don't like to use the word **'diet'** when discussing weight loss or muscle gain, as it implies a reduction or increased consumption of calories.

This has been buried deeply in the psyche of the nation, and gives the wrong impression to what I prefer to call..."**Weight management**".
Let's get started by first looking at the two ways in, which you can combat an overweight problem...

** *The first one is to lower your calorie intake to a level of starvation*

In my opinion, this is the biggest mistake most dieters make when starting a diet, they lower their calorie intake far too much, in some cases over 2000+ calories a day.

This can only ever result in the dieter starving themselves to a point, when they are forced to give up, and end up putting on even more weight.

** *The second way is to reduce your calorie intake by only 200 calories a day*

This will keep you way above the level that starvation begins, at the same time you will be able to exercise to burn off excess calories.

In this way not only do you avoid the feeling of starving, but you also tone-up the muscles and increase your fitness.

Tip: Remember this, burn it into your psyche, the more muscle you have, the higher your metabolic rate will be, the higher your metabolic rate, the more fat you will burn.

If there was just one very good tip you should take away from reading this book, it's this…have a *'cheat-day'*, get off that diet, say once a week.

This is a great way to overcome the feeling of starving and rewarding yourself for sticking to your goals, being good all week. You can eat whatever you like.

There are some very sound reasons why this is a very good technique to follow.

You see, when you start a weight management programme, you start to lose weight very fast, this is usually due to water loss, but as time goes by your metabolism slows down and fewer calories and body fat get burnt.

When you have your cheat-day, the extra food intake fires up the metabolism again, this burns off the extra calorie intake, but it doesn't stop there.

Because this new acceleration of the metabolism (fat burning) continues on for at least 48 hours, or more, wasting fat.

So, long after burning away the extra calorie intake it also goes on to burn off the stubborn body fat…you lose weight faster.

Bodybuilders have know this for decades, and have used this particular technique when preparing for a competition show.

It's not unusual to see bodybuilder's drop their body fat levels down to as low as **4%**… showing no fat or water over their muscles.

This takes a lot of knowledge of how the body works and the tricks they have to use in order to achieve these levels.

I, and other competitors noticed that after a bodybuilding competition, when we started to eat lots of cakes and chocolates again, on the following day we look even more... **RIPPED**!

Okay, if you are not a bodybuilder, then you could skip this section and move on to page 13 - *Just How Much Should You Eat to lose or gain muscle mass?*

But there is also a lot of very useful information, which you may find of interest, in this section, which may also help in your quest to lose weight.

So 'Why' is Building Big, Hard, and Chiselled Like Abs so Important to Men

There have been many studies carried out to try and answer this question.

Some recent studies as shown that **32%** of women rate abs, has the sexiest muscle group in man, but 'Why'? When you think about it just how many times do you see a men's ads, not in the night club, or when he is walk down the high street, or at work?

But a study carried out last year show that **60%** of women were turned on by the size of a man's neck and shoulders?

I guess that the neck and shoulders are more visible than abs, but still there's a lot to be said about the overall package.

Believe it or not, but the size of your guns (arms) are more important to men.

The bigger someone's arms look, the more impressed men seem to be.

I suspect that this as something to do with man's primeval instinct, big arms are more of a threat, you wouldn't like to be hit by someone with big arms.

To help you understand **'How'** your body works the following tips may be helpful:

The Best Way to Reveal Your Six-Pack

Many confuse losing weight with seeing their six-pack, but losing any weight for some, isn't easy, and running around in the dark is going to get you nowhere.

Many people are also very confused when it comes to the best way to train their abs.
Sometimes the word being spread around the gym isn't entirely accurate.

Here are four of the most common misconceptions most people have about training their abs.

MYTH 1: Abs needs to be trained every day?

Would you train your chest, arms, or shoulders every day? Then why do the same with your abs? To develop chiselled abs, they need to be trained no more than once every two days. Your abs need rest and recovery, just like any other muscle group.

MYTH 2: High reps will burn the fat from my stomach?

Doing millions of crunches will develop flat-looking abs... I don't think so?

It will, however, build endurance. I know 100's of people in the Martial Arts, who can do 1000's of sit-ups, but they don't have big abs, and in many cases they carry quite a lot of body fat, so you can't even see their abs.

For the chiselled look, you need some kind of abdominal exercise that provides resistance (such as sit-ups on an incline board, or weighted crunches).

MYTH 3: You can train the upper and lower abs separately?

The notion that you can train your upper abs using sit-ups, and your lower abs with leg raises, for example, simply isn't true.

While these exercises may seem to EMPHASISE one area of your Abdominal, your lower and upper abs (as they are often mistakenly called) are all one muscle.

For most people, the lower and upper abs can't be isolated from each other.

MYTH 4: You can spot-reduce fat from your love handles, your lower stomach, or anywhere you like?

This is probably the biggest and most miss understood myth of them all.

People really do believe that it's possible to spot reduce fat from just any part of their stomach or love handles.

Unfortunately, this couldn't be further from the truth, because as fat goes on - it will come off, or, first on, last off.

In other words, it's impossible to spot reduce fat.

Fat is deposited around the love handles first, then the stomach, then spreads up and down the body.

To lose fat this process will have to be reversed and the first place fat build-up occurs becomes the last place it disappears.

Abdominal muscles are no different to any other muscles in your body and this is why most people fail to capitalize on building abs, because they treat them as if they were a different muscle type.

You should train your abs with weights, holding a weight on your chest and doing crunches or holding a dumbbell between your feet whilst doing leg raises, will help build strong, deep, chiselled abs.

Another big mistake many people make is doing high repetitions, and then training them every day?

Ab muscles need rest just like any other muscle in your body, deny them rest, and they just won't grow. If however, you are training them for endurance, say boxing, for example, then by all mains, do high reps.

There are two distinct ways to affect good looking abs

First, reduce fat through doing cardiovascular exercise (CV for short). The aim is to raise your heart beat and maintain this rate for a prolonged period of time.

This can be done on the treadmill, crossover, steps, exercise bike, rower, or boxing bags.

Fitness is a measure of how quickly your heart beat returns to its normal or resting rate.

Secondly, is to directly train the abs through crunches, leg raises with weights.

But without a doubt, doing both of the above exercises will help accelerate the fat burning process; it will make you feel more energized, healthy, and alert.

Muscle burns "fat"

Having, or, enquiring more muscle mass, is arguably the single most important factor determining how many calories your body will burn.

This is, because your muscle is the most metabolically active tissue in the body.

Thus the more muscle you maintain, the more fat burning furnaces you will have to help you burn off those calories - even at rest.

When is it the best time to train

If you are looking to lose weight, then the best time to train is in the morning on an empty stomach.

This is, because, the body burns off stored fat rather than the calories you eat for your breakfast.

Training in the morning raises the metabolism for the rest of the day. Train no more than three times a week.

But, the most important thing to bear in mind is this, a six-pack isn't made in the gym; it's made in the kitchen.

I have known many people over the last 40 years I've been involved in bodybuilding, who worked-out hard, then go down the pub.

This puts back all the calories they have just burnt off in the gym, it's no wonder they will never see their six-pack.

The fact remains that if you want to reduce your body fat then you are going to have to increase your exercise, or reduce your calorie intake.

A good diet that containing enough high-quality protein (such as chicken, beef, and fish).

And moderate amounts of unrefined carbohydrate, and plenty of healthy fats (found in salmon, mackerel, or flaxseed oil), is the best way to strip away the fat, and reveal your abdominal muscles.

Let's start this fascinating journey into weight management, by taking a look at the evidence and its effects:

But first you will need to work out just how many calories you will need to consume just to maintain your bodyweight.

Without this information, you can't move forward.

Just How Much Should You Eat to lose Fat or gain muscle mass

It's very easy to say *'Eat more to build muscle'* or *'Eat less to lose fat'*; this still leaves you with the question..."How Much".

If you don't know the answer to this question, you may end up cutting too many calories from your program, leaving you feeling hungry, and ready to give up. So let's first start calculating your baseline calorie number.

From this figure will be able to calculate how many calories to reduce for weight loss, or increase for mass building.

You will need a pen, paper & a calculator...

Step 1:
Write down your weight in pounds _____ X by 11 = _____
this is your <u>basic calorie needs</u>.

Step 2:
Write down you basic calorie needs_____ X Caloric cost of
your workout = _____% - This figure can be found from the
following table:

ACTIVITY LEVE	YOUR AGE
	Up to 30
Mostly sedentary	30%
Moderately active	40%
Dedicated trainner	50%
30 – 40	**40 Onwards**
25%	20%
35%	30%
	40%

(These percentages are average; as your metabolic rate
may be faster or slower)

This will = _____ Your <u>metabolic rate</u>

Step 3:

Write down your basic calorie needs _____ + Your metabolic rate _____ = _____ Your <u>maintenance total</u>.

This sum reveals how many calories you need to just maintain your current body weight without losing or gaining any muscle mass.

Step 4:

How write down your maintenance total _____ + 500 = _____ To gain muscle.

Or

Step 5:

Your maintenance total _____ - 500 = _____ to lose body fat.

A pound of fat = 3,500 calories, so if you increase by 500 calories per day then you will gain 1 pound for body weight per week.

And if you reduce by 500 calories per day then you will lose 1 pound of body fat per week.

You first need to make up your mind as to what it is you want to achieve and then set out your goals, do the above calculations to find your baseline, and get going.

So what foods are good or bad for you? Study the tables below to find out

Just a thought...you know you wouldn't put anything, but petrol into a petrol car, anything else and the engine wouldn't run. But human beings throw almost anything down their throats and then complain when it goes wrong.

Treat your body in the same way you would treat an expensive car, remember, you can replace a car, but not your body; it's yours for... **'Life'**!

PROTEIN

Bad Foods	Because
Beef or Pork Ribs Brisket Ground Beef Pork Sausages	They are very high in saturated fats, which are linked to heart disease – and, because it goes down so fast that your body doesn't have the time to achieve its appetite – controlling mechanism.

Except for these foods they are better for you

Eggs

Fish, including water-packed canned tuna.

Lean cuts of meat such as Sirloin, Flank, or Tenderloin.

90% ground Beef or Turkey, chewed slowly.

Reduced-fat lunchmeats (Roast Beef, Turkey, Ham).

Skinless Chicken or Turkey breast.

Turkey – Sausage

STARCHES

Bad Foods	**Because**
Pasta Potatoes Sugar-laden or low-fibre breakfast cereals. White bread White rice	Quickly digested, leaving you feeling hungry soon after. It's best to eat a carbohydrate that's packed with some fibre, backed potato for example; fibre is linked to lower heart disease.

Except for these foods they are better for you

If eaten immediately before or after exercise. Should be combined with good protein such as eggs or low-fat dairy products.	Rye bread Sweet potatoes. Whole grain bread, pasta, rice. Whole-wheat pitas. All-bran. Grape-nuts. Oatmeal. Raisin bran. Shredded Wheat – Shredded Wheat 'N Bran'.

DAIRY

Bad Foods   Because

Whole mike and other full-fat dairy products	Because they are high in saturated fat and/or Transit fats...the most deadliest known

Except for these foods they are better for you

	Skimmed milk or fat-free milk. Or other dairy products that are no more than 2 to 1% fat content. Like cottage cheese.

FRUITS

Bad Foods   Because

Dried fruit such as raisins and prunes.	It's far too easy to eat too many calories at any one sitting.

Except for these foods they are better for you

Apples.	Oranges
Bananas	Pears
Blackberries	Plums
Blueberries	Raspberries
Cherries	Strawberries
Grapefruit	Kiwifruit

VEGETABLES

Bad Foods	Because
Carrots Corn	Relatively high in sugar but low in nutrients.

Except for these foods they are better for you

Asparagus	Mushrooms
Avocado	Onions
Broccoli	Peas
Brussels sprouts	Peppers
Cauliflower	Spinach
Eggplant	Tomatoes
Green beans	Zucchini
Lettuce (the darker, the better)	

NUTS & SEEDS

Bad Foods	Because
Macadamia nuts	

Except for these foods they are better for you

Peanuts (Its technically a vegetable, but usually included in this category)	Almonds Brazil nuts Pecans Sunflower seeds Walnuts

SNACKS

Bad Foods	Because
Chips Pretzels	Even low-fat chips are nothing more than extra carbohydrates, if laden with salt this will cause your body to retain water, making your body look fatter.

Except for these foods they are better for you

When at a party, if you dip your chips into guacamole, then you will at least be eating monounsaturated fats…the same good fat as found in olive oil.	Apples, Peanut butter, string cheese. These foods may contain many calories, but they contain the proteins and fats that will help to make you feel fuller for longer.

FATS AND OILS

Bad Foods   Because

Bad Foods	Because
Butter	High in saturated fat
Coconut oil	High in trans fats, thought to be more unhealthy than saturated fats
Margarine	
Vegetable shortening	

Except for these foods they are better for you

Used in a cautiously way, butter can turn a slice of whole grain toast into a decent snack, since it's appetizing and the fat helps you feel fuller longer. The fibre in the whole grain bread is good too.	Benecol spread Canola oil Flaxseed oil Olive oil Peanut oil Sesame oil Smart Balance spread Corn oil

Note: Corn oil is high in omega-6 fatty acids. You need Fatty acids, which are very good for you, but you should include omega 3 & 9 along with omega-6.

BEVERAGES

Bad Foods	Because
Apple juice Flavoured ice tea Juice drinks Soda	Apple juice is high in fructose, which doesn't generate an insulin response. Meaning it won't shut off your appetite, it's stored as fat. Most sodas are sweetened with high fructose com syrups

Except for these foods they are better for you

	Coffee (in limited amounts) Crystal light Diet soda Herbal tea Pure fruit juice Tea Unsweetened seltzer Water

The basic rule of thumb when dieting is to make sure that you get enough calories to fuel your life-style, or training session.

Most bodybuilders up their percentage of protein, and that's right, because, protein builds and repairs muscles.

But if you don't eat enough carbohydrates then your body will convert a percentage of your protein intake into fuel.

This is not a good idea, because you will endup leaving too little protein to carry out the basic body repairs, you will, in fact, find yourself in a losing position.

And if you don't eat enough protein, your body will cannibalize fuel from the stores of carbohydrates in your muscles, and your muscles will decrease in size.

But should you eat too much clean protein (Chicken, fish, etc.), don't worry, because your body will pass it out, and will not store it as fat.

But a note of warning, if you don't curb the amounts of carbohydrates you eat then the excess 'will' get stored as fat.

Tip: 1. if you are trying to lose weight, then do your training first thing in the morning, on an empty stomach, this will help to accelerate fat loss.

Don't eat, for about one hour after training, because your body will continue to burn fat at an accelerated rate.

Tip: 2. if you body-build then eat your first meal as soon as you get up in the morning, one of the best meals you can start the day are 'oats', they release energy slowly during the day.

Eat small meals every 3 – 4 hours.

Have a pre-meal snack or drink about an hour before training, and then have a protein drink straight after you have finished, within 30minutes of ending your session.

Your body will absorb ALL this extra protein to start the repair process.

Tip: 3. if you feel a little peckish then reach for a packet of mixed nuts. They are full of protein, essential oils and fibre; it's recommended that you eat about two hand full's daily.

Supplements

The subject of taking supplements is huge, and I can't do it full justice here, but they are vitally important for anyone who is embarking on a weight loss and control management program.

They are so important I'm going to give you a brief summery of all the vitamins, and minerals, you need to take in order to keep a fully functional body.

All over our globe there are lots of people having problems with their digestive systems, which make it hard to absorb nutrients and break down the food they eat.

This is a common problem, one that is usually caused by a poor level of acid in the stomach, toxicants in the gut, or a decrease, in the production of enzymes that assist with the food breakdown process.

Nutrients and vitamins are highly important for your health; a diet that is high in organic matter is the preferred way to improve your digestion, although you may need to use supplements as well.

The best thing about supplements is the fact that you don't need a prescription. You can select which ones you want on your own, and purchase them at your local nutrition store or online.

Vitamins that are water soluble are the easiest to use, as they will pass through the body easily and quickly, and should be taken three times a day.

Vitamins that are fat soluble are best absorbed if they are taken with food that contains fat. The ideal time to take supplements is with your meals.

Below, is a list of the most common vitamins you should consider taking and how to take them:

** **Vitamins A, D, and E** - These vitamins should always be taken with meals that contain fat or oil.

** **Vitamin B** - You should always take vitamin B supplements as soon as you wake up, to get the maximum benefit. You can also take them during the day with a whole grain meal.

** **Vitamin C** - Supplements containing vitamin C should be taken with meals and never on an empty stomach.

** **Iron** - Iron supplements should always be taken with food, as they are easier to absorb this way.

** **Multi-vitamins** -You can take multi-vitamins at anytime, although you should always consume a small meal with the supplement.

Even though you may be on a healthy diet, you should still make sure that you are getting the proper vitamins and supplements as well.

If you include supplements in your diet and take them correctly, you'll find that your body will be much healthier, and will respond better to your new lifestyle.

A Weight Management Programme We All Should Follow

I've been to Greece and to Tuscany in Italy, and for those who haven't; I can tell you that their Mediterranean cuisine is fabulous.

They are full of richly coloured heart-healthy fruits, vegetables, whole grains, fish and poultry and, of course, plenty of olive oil...fascinating, **'Why'**?

Because, in spite of the liberal use of oils and grains, researchers have found that people who eat a ***"Mediterranean type diet"***, have vastly lower rates of heart disease, than people in many other parts of the world.

Dimitrios Trichopoulos, MD, Ph.D., from the Harvard School of Public Health, worked with a group of Greek scientists from the University Of Athens Medical School, to investigate the impact of their diet.

For the study...22,000 Greek men and women, ages 20 to 86, recorded what they ate each day over a four-year period.
The investigators then rated their responses, on a scale of zero through to 10, based on how closely the participants stayed with the tenets of the diet, with 10 being the best.

They discovered that following the diet, not only lowered the risk of death by heart disease, or stroke, but that for every two-point increase achieved in the rating scale, there was a **25%** drop in mortality risk.

A separate, but similar American study showed that the diet also helps reduce the risk of gallstones, by nearly 20%.

Let's look at these dietary details. Unlike the detailed approach of many weight-loss plans, this diet has no particular structure.

The Mediterranean diet includes...

** Lots of fruits and vegetables
** Plenty of whole-grain products
** Some beans, legumes and nuts
** A moderate amount of fish and poultry
** Limited amounts of meats, dairy and alcohol.

Dr. Rimm offers the following strategies for sticking with a true, Mediterranean diet...

Whole grains are whole grains

In addition to their nutritive value, whole grains slow the digestion of other foods, leaving you feeling fuller for a longer period of time.

This lowers the **"Net-crab"** effect. He urges people to select the least processed whole-grain foods, even if, a food is technically a whole grain.

Any commercial preparation, or images, of those fabulous fresh breads, can get you thinking; whether pulverizing the grain will reduce its healthiness... don't be fooled by these packaging ploys.

Bread, for example, must have the word **"whole"** as its first or, second ingredient, listed on its ingredients list, to qualify as truly whole wheat.

Variety of grain

Sure this is the mainstay of the Mediterranean's, but in fact they eat a variety of delicious and nutritious grains. Brown rice also counts, as do a number of other grain products, including oats (especially steel-cut oats), and barley.

Lots of vegetables

The Greeks typically eat nearly a pound of vegetables a day! Twice what Americans eat? Don't be shy with your vegetables.

Plenty of protein

I advise you to keep your protein clean (no junk food), on a daily basis, be it fish, poultry or eggs. Plant protein, in the form of beans and nuts, also is good...just what the dieter ordered!

Counting calories

Portion control is always going to be your watchword, even when it comes to consuming olive oil.

Although the Mediterranean diet features up to **40%** of calories from fat, this includes all sources, including fish, poultry and dairy, as well as from monounsaturated oils, like canola, soy, and especially olive oil.

"Super-sizing"

your portion definitely is not the way to go. Eat small amounts, throughout the day.

Active lifestyle

Another critical aspect of Mediterranean eating is their way of life.

Exercise is as much a part of their diet, as is olive oil. These people work hard physically, each day, unlike Americans, who live a more sedentary life.

It's mandatory to get at least 30 minutes of brisk exercises a day, most days.

You should limit other *"extra"* foods to occasional treats; these foods include red meats, unless you are a bodybuilder, which are tolerable only a couple of times a week.

Even then think small, don't binge on three scoops of ice cream. The diet includes dairy, but doesn't emphasize it. Stick with low-fat products when possible, and limit portions.

Although the above diet will help those who are looking to reduce their overall weight, don't be fooled into believing that it has no value for those looking to increase muscle size neither.

Because, following the basic outline of this diet, will help you achieve your goals.

Now I hear you asking... well muscle also requires more than just proteins?

They also require, good fats, minerals and vitamins, to help stimulate muscle growth, well guess what, 'yes' this diet does just that.

First, make the decision and set it as a goal. Over whatever period of time you are comfortable with, slide the right foods into your eating regimen and the wrong ones out.

We are all different and require different mixes of management, so review often and see what changes you may need to make.

Just remember to increase your proteins and bob's your uncle... job done.

A Rule of Thumb

There is a rule that you can follow regardless of whether you are trying to lose or gain weight.

You should be eating, around 5-6 small meals a day.

'Yes' I know, this sounds like a lot of food when you're trying to lose weight, but remember what I was saying about the average diet that hit the high streets, a whopping **95%** of those people who go on a diet will...**'fail'**.

You must learn how your body works, if it's not getting enough calories, your body will respond by going into what we call **'Starvation mould'**, and will hang on to every calorie you eat, converting it into fat.

By eating more food and I mean, good clean foods, may-be a little bad food like crisps, chocolate etc, but just now and again, will trick your body into not slipping into starvation mould.

You also need to understand, that our body's temperature rises, in response to the digestion of food; this in turn burns calories at a higher rate.

When our metabolic rate increases this is known as **'Thermogenesis'**.

Now stop, and think about this for a minute, your body temperature rises every time you eat, for this reason alone eating *5-6 small meals a day*, as got to be worth it.

Because, eating more good food will help speed up your metabolism, reducing body fat, and increasing your energy.

If you are trying to lose weight, then **'Don't'** reduce your calorie intake by too much, this is the biggest mistake most people make.

They tend to decrease their calorie intake by 1000 calories, or more, a day, and then give up, because, they are starving.

And even more disturbing for the bodybuilder, this course of action will lead to lower energy levels, muscle deterioration, or shrinkage, and a slower metabolic rate.

Remember that your body works on a priority system, the first priority being **'Survival'**!

And when you go on a **'Diet'** it doesn't know you are dieting, it thinks you are starving, so it makes you feel hungry.

Hunger is nothing more than a protective mechanism set-up to keep us alive, and nothing more.

In fact, there are times when hunger strikes, even when your body doesn't really require any food, it's simply reminding you to eat.

This maybe, because you can smell food, or you reach for food in order to help heal psychological hurts, loneliness, anger, anxiety, for example.

Learn to recognize, which hunger signs you are receiving. You will know real hunger, when you feel hunger pains, these represent the only true hunger feelings you should respond to.

Instead, reduce your daily calorie intake, by 200 calories a day, then stick with it, for about 'four' weeks.

If you don't start to reduce weight, then reduce your calorie intake by another 200 calories a day. When you do start to lose these unwanted pounds, stop, don't reduce any further.

If on the other hand, you start to lose too much weight, too quickly, then increase your calorie intake, by 100 calories at a time, until you find a balance that allows you to lose weight.

And then, and this is important, just maintain that calorie intake…remember that you don't want to lose any muscle size.

Another problem, I would like to quickly address

When people embark on their diets, they have this tendency to concentrate on the amount of weight they lose, instead of the amount of fat, which is what they are trying to lose.

You see, when you go on any diet, you will first start to lose weight, through water, and muscle removal, and last of all…fat.

This leads to people becoming dependant on using their bathroom scales to judge their weight loss, it becomes a compulsion to constantly check their body weight with their scales.

This isn't a very good indicator of weight loss, because when you diet your body will constantly adjust itself to fit its new situation.

So one minute you will be weighing lighter, and the next, heavier.

This constant change gives you the wrong impression, leading to confusion and disappointment; you should however, endeavour to use the mirror, and go by what you see.

In fact when going on a high street diet, you can lose up to **50%** of your weight, from lean body mass; your muscles are being used for food by your starving body, and for anyone who trains hard, that's the last thing they want.

How to count your calories

At first, counting calories may seem weird, or out of place, but after a short while, it will become second nature to you.

Each of the food items you eat should show the calorie count on the container label.

For instance, a cup of skimmed milk is 90 calories, and it says so right on the back of the carton. A serving of whey protein is 120 calories.

Each meal must, and I repeat, must, contain a balance of protein, complex carbohydrates. White bread, white rice, and sugars, for example, are simple carbs, and will release quickly into your blood stream.

Whereas, proteins contain fats (the fatty acid type), and complex carbohydrates, brown rice, brown bread, oats, etc., will release more slowly into your bloodstream, giving you a constant flow of energy.

Divide your calories up into six meals a day. So if you were, for example, to consume say, 2,400 calories a day, each of your meals would be approximately 400 calories each...get the idea.

A great meal would be a turkey sandwich, for example, or a lean piece of steak, with oven baked sweet potatoes.

The carbohydrate should be a complex one, such as oatmeal or whole wheat bread; your protein should be from a low-fat source.

In other words, cut out the bacon and ribs from your diet, and adopt, lean turkey, lean steak, and lean chicken.

You should also try to eat all your calories in-between the hours of waking and midday. In this way, your body will burn up those calories over the course of the day.

Reduce the calorie content of your meals as the day goes by, and make your last meal a purely protein one…absolutely 'No' carbs.

Note: If you are looking to increase muscle size, then increase both your calorie and protein intake, but remember to do this slowly, as you need to find a balance, that will allow you to increase muscle size without the body fat.

Unfortunately, there really isn't any way around this dilemma, unless you have the perfect genetics.

If you are eating too many calories for the amount of fuel you are burning off during everyday activity, or exercise, then you will put on body fat.

And if you don't eat enough calories, then you won't put on any real muscle mass, you will simply, end-up losing water and muscle. You also run the risk of fatiguing your body…the trick is to find a *balance*.

Now, before we leave this subject of **'Diets'**, let me show you a very sound reason **'Why'**, you should consider reducing your calories, even if you are not looking to lose weight?

Reduce Calories for Your Heart's Sake

Even if you aren't interested in losing weight or increasing muscle size, there is good evidence to suggest, a well-balanced diet, as some very welcome benefits, for us all.

For decades now, health professionals have believed that those who eat less tend to live longer; a study recently released by the University of Wisconsin, offers even more support for this belief.

Researchers measured how caloric intake affects heart function, and came to the conclusion that less food could possibly result in a healthier heart.

Based on their finding, it appears that if people reduce their current calorie intake, between 20 and **40%**, even starting in middle age, they may delay the development of heart disease, or possibly even prevent it.

According to professor of genetics Tomas Prolla, Ph.D., when hearts get older, the cells change their source of energy, from fat molecules, to carbohydrate molecules.

Carbohydrate molecules are burned at a faster rate, which leaves the heart with less energy to perform its function.

In effect, the heart becomes stressed out; this is the first step leading to heart failure.

But, when Prolla's team reduced the calorie intake of mice, the change in energy source was seen less in those who maintained a normal calorie intake.

So don't be afraid to reduce your calorie intake, you could live longer, happier, lives.

You Need 'Water' to lose weight

There is **NO**, scientific evidence, to show that drinking water will reduce fat levels.

But I have given this subject some special mention, because of its importance.

During any weight management programme, it's absolutely vital to never ignore the need to consume more water (about 4 pints a day).

Becoming hydrated, this is the point where your body as reached its ideal water levels, helps your body store glycogen (blood sugar), and directly affects all your metabolic functions.

This includes your ability to train hard, and cool down, during your workout.

Thirst, is not a good indicator of need, thirst is indeed, an indication that your body may already be very low on water, which may be enough to seriously impair performance.

So don't wait until you feel thirsty, sip water during your workout, it's so important.

Also, drink water before a meal, but don't drink it straight from the fridge.

Research has shown that drinking cold water will slow down your metabolism, a process by, which food is converted into energy; you need to drink it at room temperature.

If, on the other hand, you are looking to increase bodyweight, then you should drink it cold.

Apart from water you need 'Sleep' Too

Believe it or not, but not getting eight hours of sleep a night, can decrease your chances of losing weight?

Sleep deprivation is on the increase, and whilst eight hours of work, eight hours of play, and eight hours of sleep, used to represent the magic triangle of balance in a person's life, now, sleeping cycles are becoming shorter.

You should strive to get seven, or more, hours of sleep per night, or you risk perturbations in your hormone levels…like growth hormone (GH).

GH peaks in the middle of your sleep, and is responsible for repairing, and producing new cells, throughout your body.

If you don't get enough deep sleep, then you run the risk of fatigue.

Important note, studies have conclusively shown, that those who routinely get less than eight hours sleep a night, tend to gain more…body fat!

Essential Fatty Acids – You Need Them

Some fats, called essential fatty acids, are a key component to trigger unlimited metabolic growth.

Essential fatty acids are required to manufacture a whole bunch of growth producing hormones.

When you eat nutritious fats, you body will be able to flood your system with testosterone and growth hormone.

Fats are also an easy and convenient way, to crank up your calories, big time.

Again, if it grows, eat it…avocadoes, nuts, olives, organic peanut butter, etc.

Bottled oils can be extremely powerful such as evening primrose oil, hemp oil or extra virgin olive oil.

These are all excellent sources of essential fatty acids.

Not all fats are created equal, in-fact, most of the fats found today, such as margarine, cheeses, (except cottage cheese), red meat, fried foods, and many hidden fats found in packaged food, are totally detrimental to your health and to building big muscles.

These fats will clog up your system and make you fat…fast.

A good rule of thumb to remember is: If it is heated - we do not eat it.

Bad fat's breakdown when subjected to heat, they become rancid, creating trans-fatty acids, which are to be avoided at all costs.

Also, do not eat fats that harden at room temperature, because your body cannot digest these fats easily, or, effectively.

Green Tea Stimulates Fat Burning

There are now many studies reporting the health benefits, of green tea extract.

In particular, studies had pointed to the potential of green tea extract to enhance fat oxidation.

Japanese researchers have further contributed to this line of research, by assessing the metabolic effects of green tea, during exercise.

Green tea, is very bitter to drink, so why not combined the fantastic benefits of taking Honey, with the benefits of consuming green tea?

Simply add it to your green tea, to help make it sweeter…enjoy!!

Can you have Carbohydrates after your training

In a recent study, scientists gave subjects a protein and carbohydrate supplement, either immediately following, or three hours after exercise.

The results show, that muscle growth was far greater when the supplement was taken immediately after exercise, compared to, when it was taken 3 hours later.

Tip: You should take a protein drink within 30 – 45 minutes after training.

An important note for those who are trying to burn body fat... When you train you deplete your muscles of glucose, and up to 30 minutes after training, you can eat as many carbohydrates, and proteins as you want,

Your body will **NOT** lay down any of these calories as body fat. This is a trick bodybuilders have been using for years to get their body fat levels down to **4%**, way below that of the average dieter.

So don't be afraid to consume protein drinks that contain a high level of carbohydrates.

Whey protein drinks are an excellent source of protein, and carbohydrates, because, they are absorbed very quickly by the body.

Solid food, on the other hand, would take far too long to be absorbed by the body, missing the window of opportunity.

It's important to know how the body works, and in particular, how 'your' body works, no two people are the same.

There's only one way in, which you can find this out, and that's by experimentation.

Follow the guide-lines, outlined above, and be prepared to adjust as time goes by, and you will see success.

My Biggest Tip or Hidden Secret, to Permanently Keeping Off Your Weight is...

Have a... 'Cheat-Day'!

'Yes', eat and indulge in your favourite 'Cheat' foods like delicious burgers, pizza, ice cream and cakes, on one day per week and NEVER store the extra calories as fat?

You see, when you first go on any calorie reduced diet, you lose weight very fast.

But as time ebbs by, your metabolism starts to slowdown, and losing any weight just gets harder.

So having a 'Cheat-day', fully firesup your metabolism again, but it doesn't end there.

Because, this action of firing up the metabolism lasts for several days, it continues to not only burn off the extra calories you eat on your cheat day, but it goes on to burn off the 'Stubborn' fat too.

This is not only a excellent way to give yourself a treat for staying on target, and reaching your goals, but it *STOPS* you from feeling hungry all of the time.

This will dramatically reduce any feelings of starvation, pecking away at your willpower to stay the course.

And the bonus, the reduction of stubborn body fat too!

Enjoy your 'Cheat Day'... and lose weight for life!

Conclusion

1.   Remember, that the high street diet will lower your metabolism, and you should   do every-thing in your power to avoid doing this.

To help keep your metabolism rate high, follow the recommended tips above.

2.   Intense, short, exercise sessions, is an excellent way to increase your metabolism rate.

'High Intensity Training' (HIT) workouts, puts greater demands upon your body, which in turn, forces the body to burn more food faster.   Thus greater fat loss and muscle growth.

3.   You must not starve your body, eat more, but smaller meals throughout the day; about 5 to 6 meals a day should be your target food intake, about 3 hours apart.

4.   Do some type of cardiovascular activity, at least three times a week, to higher your heart rate?

This type of activity will burn off more calories, exercise the heart and lungs, increase blood flow, and oxygen to your muscles.

You will feel fitter, more active, and an increase in your sense of well-being.

5.   Have a *'Cheat day'*, and Stop your cravings for food, reduce stubborn fat, kick start your metabolism, and reward yourself for reaching your goals... build a fat-free lifestyle!

Supplements to help you lose fat

There are a number of very good supplements, designed to help you lose body fat. I can recommend two very good supplements, which I have used myself:

** *SidaCordifolia* (400mg 900 capsules)

This is an **excellent fat burner**, which is also used to boost energy levels.

SidaCordifolia, is a natural herb, which stimulates the body's nervous system to produce more energy.

For more info go to - http://increasemusclesize.net/sida-cordifolia

** *Rhodiola Rosea* (90 Capsules)

Strengthens the nervous system, fights depression, enhances immunity, and elevates the capacity for exercise, enhances memory, **aids weight reduction**, increase sexual functions and improves energy levels.

For more info go to - http://increasemusclesize.net/rhodiola-rosea

To learn more about what supplements and vitamins are all available, how they work, and what makes a good, bad, or, down-right ugly supplement, copy this link...
http://increasemusclesize.net/?p=942

These an old saying that goes something like this...**"You are what you eat"**, and guess what, it's absolutely true.

I have shown you a way in, which it's possible to 'beat' and manage your weight problem, but now the time has come to stop, **"Talking the talk"**, and start...**"Walking the walk"**.

It's up to you, you have to make a decision now.

But remember, whatever decision you make now, will affect you for the rest of your life. If you have decided to get with the program and lose weight... remember it's for life.

My message to you is ...*'It's the life-style you lead, that will determine your outcome'*.

All that is left for me to say is... *"All my best wishes in all your future endeavours, I hope you find inner peace"!*

Judge J

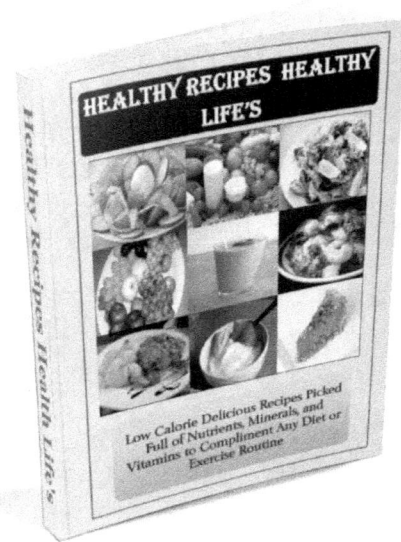

Further reading...

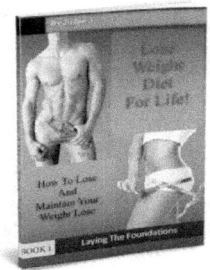

Now that you have a deeper understanding of what needs to put into place, in order to achieve your final weight loss goals. You now need to build that all important and essential support network, and foundation, to keep you on the straight and narrow, read my **1st** book...'Lose Weight Diet For Life'!

If you are adamant about going straight onto a diet without first understanding the need for a rock solid foundation, then you are asking to fail. It's important to lay down a supportive foundation right from the word go. Diets are by their very nature stressful and demanding on the body and if you have no safety net in place, failure will be your only reward.

A solid foundation is a fundamental part of the overall strategy when losing weight. If you have ever found it hard to lose, or, keep off weight, then don't miss out reading this very important step. To find out more about what this book as to offer, or to grab your own *copy* *visit:*
http://mybooksupply.com/wp/lose-weight-diet-for-life

*If you enjoy my work, please feel free to visit my **Website** at:*
http://mybooksupply.com

'Twitter': @hotwealth
'LinkedIn': *http://uk.linkedin.com/in/judgej*
'Facebook': *https://www.facebook.com/pages/Lose-weight-manage-weight/343091449182861*

CONTENTS...